Addicting Medications
No Functional Recovery
The Long View
Your Nineteenth Psychiatric Consultation
William R. Yee M.D., J.D.
Applied for December 12th, 2020

I have been practicing general medicine, emergency room medicine, and psychiatry since 1972 without interruption in Michigan, Indiana, Kentucky, California and Texas.

My experience since 1970 is that addicting medications provide a temporary and marginal benefit that dissipates with addiction.

After the addiction, pain, insomnia, and anxiety are worse than when the patient was first treated. This is clearly demonstrated during withdrawal from medications and alcohol used for anxiety, pain, and insomnia.

During withdrawal the brain is hyperactive to the point of seizure and the pain, anxiety, and insomnia manifest in their most extreme forms.

If the reader has not been exposed to drug and alcohol withdrawal, I suggest watching videos of DT's and drug withdrawal on YouTube.

Prior to exposure to addicting medications patients do not display anxiety, pain, or insomnia that comes close to what they face when they stop using addicting medications for the use of anxiety, pain and insomnia.

My practice of medicine and psychiatry has always been evidenced based.

By that, I mean I would read the Physician's Desk Reference, (PDR), and the available literature before prescribing psychotropic medications, (medications used to treat mental illness).

My practice of medicine and psychiatry has been grounded in a college education that included, calculus, chemistry, organic chemistry, biology, embryology, physics, psychology, social anthropology, and a medical school education that included biochemistry, human anatomy that required that I spend a year dissecting a human body with three lab partners, physiology, pathology, genetics, psychiatry, internal medicine, dermatology, radiology, emergency room medicine, surgery, obstetrics/gynecology, pediatrics, among other courses.

I found surgery to be the most rigorous and disciplined of the rotations while in medical school.

The most impressive parts of the surgery rotation were the Friday afternoon morbidity and mortality rounds.

During morbidity and mortality rounds the professors, residents and interns reviewed all the surgical cases with complications and death.

The course of diagnosis and treatments from admissions to discharges were reviewed.

The complications were examined for causes, treatments, and outcomes.

All the currently available alternative treatments were examined from the perspective of risks and benefits.

After this was done, there was a discussion of what the best practice was in each case.

After a best practice was identified, that became the best practice for the future by all the surgeons, residents and interns in the department of surgery.

There was no discussion of fault or blame.

The focus was on finding the causes of the complications and the best practice to minimize complications and deaths in the future.

This strategy became part of my thinking for the past fifty years.

I monitor treatments and outcomes in every case and consider alternatives for the best practice.

From time to time, I review the literature to ascertain if my practice is the best practice.

This book is a product of my continuing effort to provide the best care based upon the current evidence available in the medical literature.

Finding the best practice is not a simple matter when reviewing the literature.

Research in medicine and the use of psychotropic medications is rife with flaws that create errors.

First there is publication bias.

For a fact check and deeper look I refer the reader to:

Publication bias in meta-analyses from the Cochrane Database of Systematic Reviews
Michal Kicinski, David A. Springate, Evangelos Kontopantelis
First published: 18 May 2015
https://doi.org/10.1002/sim.6525

For more information I refer the reader to:
From Wikipedia, the free encyclopedia:
"Not to be confused with Reporting bias or Media bias."

"Publication bias is a type of bias that occurs in published academic research. It occurs when the outcome of an experiment or research study influences the decision whether to publish or otherwise distribute it. Publishing only results that show a significant finding disturbs the balance of findings and inserts bias in favor of positive results.[1] The study of publication bias is an important topic in metascience."

"Studies with significant results can be of the same standard as studies with a null result with respect to quality of execution and design.[2] However, statistically significant results are three times more likely to be published than papers with null results.[3] A consequence of this is that researchers are unduly motivated to manipulate their practices to ensure that a statistically significant result is reported.[4]"

I will leave it to the reader to research the
following list of flaws in research
regarding the risks and benefits of
psychotropic medications.

Research fails to include pregnant women
and children on ethical grounds.

Research fails to include elderly and
people with multiple medical problems.

Research fails to include people on
multiple medications.

Small sample size is not sufficient to
provide reliable data.

Samples are not random because as they
do not include people who refuse to
participate.

Samples are not random because
populations may not be accessible for
research.

Studies are not randomized.

Studies are not blinded.

Studies do not use the same criteria for diagnosis or target symptoms.

The studies are of short duration.

Studies do not clearly separate spontaneous remission from medication effect.

Studies do not account for cognitive dissonance in addition to placebo effect.

It is difficult to identify altered data, "fudging."

This is not even the tip of the iceberg. One study uncovered 710 unique research flaws for excluding research from evidence-based databases.

For fact checking and a deeper look at the shortcomings of medical research I refer the reader to:

A Large-Scale Analysis of the Reasons Given for Excluding Articles that are Retrieved by Literature Search During Systematic Review

Tracy Edinger, ND, MCR and Aaron M.
Cohen, MD, MS
AMIA Annu Symp Proc. 2013; 2013: 379–
387.
Published online 2013 Nov 16.
PMCID: PMC3900186
PMID: 24551345

Let as examine the quality of medical
research in the context of scientific
research in general.

There is a crisis in scientific research.

Most research cannot be duplicated.

If the research cannot be duplicated it is
not science.

For a fact check and a deeper look, I refer
the reader to:

Sabine Hossenfelder
This is an interview with Dorothy Bishop,
Professor for Psychology at the
University of Oxford, UK. We speak about
the reproducibility crisis in psychology
and other disciplines. What is the
reproducibility crisis? How bad is it?

What can be done about it and what has been done about it?
https://www.youtube.com/watch?v=v778sv ukrtU&t=860s

At this time seventy percent, 70%, of scientific research cannot be duplicated.

For my readers who do not have access to YouTube, you can fact check and look deeper into this issue with the following:

1,500 scientists lift the lid on reproducibility
Survey sheds light on the 'crisis' rocking research.   Monya Baker
NATURE | NEWS FEATURE
25 May 2016 Corrected: 28 July 2016

In the best of all possible worlds, science should provide a guide for progress of politics, business, and social evolution. However, in the real world, politics and business corrupt science and social evolution.

The sugar industry actively redirected science, politics and social evolution from the sugar risks of obesity, diabetes and heart disease to red meat and fat.

For a fact check and a deeper look I refer the reader to :

50 Years Ago, Sugar Industry Quietly Paid Scientists To Point Blame At Fat
September 13, 20169:59 AM ET
CAMILA DOMONOSKE

and:

Sugar Industry and Coronary Heart Disease Research A Historical Analysis of Internal Industry Documents
Cristin E. Kearns, DDS, MBA1,2; Laura A. Schmidt, PhD, MSW, MPH1,3,4; Stanton A. Glantz, PhD1,5,6,7,8
Author Affiliations
JAMA Intern Med. 2016;176(11):1680-1685.
doi:10.1001/jamainternmed.2016.5394
November 2016

This was not a first, but a part of a long history of big business creating fake science to support a revenue stream.

Imagine that! Scientists being paid to create false science to influence the behavior of the public at large. Eat sugar and die? Breathe asbestos and die? Smoke cigarettes and die?

For a fact check and deeper look I refer the reader to the asbestos coverup:

Review: The Dusting of America: A Story of Asbestos: Carnage, Cover-Up, and Litigation
Reviewed Work: Outrageous Misconduct: The Asbestos Industry on Trial by Paul Brodeur
Review by: David Rosenberg
Harvard Law Review
Vol. 99, No. 7 (May, 1986), pp. 1693-1706 (14 pages)
Published By: The Harvard Law Review Association
https://doi.org/10.2307/1341085
https://www.jstor.org/stable/1341085

For a fact check and deeper look into the Tobacco Industry I refer the reader to:
Smokescreen: The Truth Behind the Tobacco Industry Cover-up
Robert N. Proctor, PhD

Author Affiliations
JAMA. 1996;276(12):998.
doi:10.1001/jama.1996.03540120076040
September 25, 1996

The pharmaceutical industry has a long record of misinformation and abuse of the marketplace. Use addicting medications and die?

For a fact check and deeper look into Neurontin/gabapentin I refer the reader to:
Pfizer to Pay $420 Million in Illegal Marketing Case, By Kenneth N. Gilpin, New York Times
May 13, 2004

For a fact check and deeper look into Oxycontin I refer the reader to:

"In May 2004, Pfizer agreed to pay $430 million and to plead guilty to criminal charges for illegally marketing Neurontin for unapproved uses such as migraine headaches and pain."

Pfizer to pay $325 million in Neurontin settlement.

By Jonathan Stempel
JUNE 2, 20149:55 AM   UPDATED 7
YEARS AGO

Regarding a fact check and a deeper look
at oxycontin I refer the reader to:

OxyContin maker Purdue Pharma pleads
guilty to criminal charges
HEALTHCARE & PHARMA
NOVEMBER 24, 2020; 12:10 PMU PDATED
12 DAYS AGO
By Mike Spector

and:

OxyContin Maker To Pay Out Billions In
Civil, Criminal Penalties
October 22, 20205:06 AM ET
LAW NPR
Heard on Morning Edition
BRIAN MAN

The Long View

In the past cocaine, laudanum and heroine were not regulated.

From Wikipedia, the free encyclopedia:

"Laudanum is a tincture (a medicine made by dissolving a drug in alcohol), of opium with about 10% powdered opium by weight (the equivalent of 1% morphine)."

According to Reddit:

"Coca-Cola contained 9 mg Cocaine in one glass of Coke until it was removed in 1903."

For a fact check and deeper look I refer the reader to:

Coca-Cola - Wikipediaen.wikipedia.org › wiki › Coca-Cola:

"Coca-Cola, or Coke, is a carbonated soft drink manufactured by The Coca-Cola Company. ... (For comparison, a typical dose or "line" of cocaine is 50–75 mg.) ..."

The pharmaceutical industry's most successful drug was Miltown.

For a fact check and deeper look I refer the reader to:

"Meprobamate—marketed as Miltown by Wallace Laboratories was one of the first drugs to be widely advertised to the general public, with user Milton Berle promoting the drug heavily on his television show, calling himself 'Uncle Miltown'.[10] Miltown soon became ubiquitous in 1950s American life, with 1 in 20 Americans having used it by late 1956"
From Wikipedia, the free encyclopedia
At one point one in twenty Americans had been treated with Meprobamate:

For a fact check and deeper look I refer the reader to:

CULTURE
America's Long Love Affair with Anti-Anxiety Drugs
BY TONY DOKOUPIL ON 1/21/09 AT 7:00 PM EST

If a doctor wishes to apply the best practice when prescribing he needs to know the risks and benefits of the medication.

One measure of the benefit is the number of patients that need to be treated for one patient to get better. This is referred to as the NNT, or Number Needed to Treat.

Another measure of the benefit is what percentage of symptoms are removed in response to the medication. The range is zero percent, 0%, to one hundred percent, 100%. Zero would be no benefit and one hundred percent would be a cure.

For psychotropic medications 20% reduction of symptoms is sufficient for the FDA to give approval for marketing the medication for the treatment of mental illness.

A 40% reduction of symptoms is a "robust," response from the point of view of the pharmaceutical industry.

The pharmaceutical industry is interested in a revenue stream and there is a great temptation to lie, steal and cheat based upon the fines and criminal prosecutions listed above.

From the viewpoint of the patient, family and significant others a cure is desired. Twenty to forty percent reduction of symptoms is not a cure.

Fifty to seventy five percent of patients stop taking psychotropic medications after eighteen months.

Is that fifty to seventy five percent properly classified as noncompliant? Or is that fifty to seventy five percent who stop taking psychotropic medications a rational vote of no confidence?

If the doctor dictates and the patient submits, then fifty to seventy five percent of the patients are noncompliant.

If the doctor informs and then the patient makes an informed choice, the fifty to seventy five percent who stop taking the medication are making a rational choice and a vote of no confidence in the medication, the FDA and the pharmaceutical industry.

The paragraph above is a sentinel event and part of boilerplate that plaintiff attorneys will use when filing summons and complaints against pharmaceutical companies, physicians, mental health centers, private clinics, peer review committees, CEO's and other entities involved in the long-term use of addicting medications generating a revenue stream.

"Noncompliant," is not politically correct.

Is it appropriate to give monthly or quarterly injections to an unwilling patient knowing that the advantage is a delay of a few months between hospital admissions?

Where is the patient's voice in the choice? This a question of ethics in view of the heavy toll of side effects including Tardive Dyskinesia that can lead to gastrotomies to allow for feeding and tracheotomies to allow for breathing.

Some patients with Tardive Dyskinesia chose suicide as a relief from cosmetic disfigurement and suffering caused by severe Tardive Dyskinesia.

There is the risk of weight gain, obesity, diabetes and poor quality of life from long term injectable antipsychotics.

Many bag ladies prefer to live on the streets as against taking medications and living in supervised facilities.

Freedom of movement and work is a current issue in the politics of the Covid-19, with worldwide demonstrations supporting the choice to move about freely and accept the risk of Covid-19.

A Deep Dive into Risks and Benefits

Having set the stage, let us take a deep dive into the use of addicting medications.

With addicting medications what are the risks and benefits?

Let us look at the risks in the context of dangerous activities such as driving a car, flying a plane or flying a helicopter.

A more demanding task is the time and attention that a mother has in caring for infants, toddlers and young children. Caring for infants, toddlers and young children is twenty-four seven and requires a continuous vigilance while monitoring children who are impulsive and likely to run in front of cars, swallow razor blades, run with knives, stick forks into electrical sockets, hide under cars, walk in front of lawn mowers, etc.

If a mother drives while sedated by sleeping pills or pain medications, she is likely to receive a ticket for impaired driving. If there are small children in the car, child protective services are likely to be called and the children may wind up in foster care for endangerment.

Pilots have lost their licenses and have been prosecuted for flying while impaired.

It is well known that people with ADHD are more likely to have car accidents than the general population. The same could be said for airplane and helicopter accidents, firearm accidents and any activity that is risky and requires vigilance does not tolerate impulsive behaviors.

For a fact check and closer look I refer the reader to the following as an entry point for more research:

Teens with ADHD get more traffic violations for risky driving, have higher crash risk
Date: May 20, 2019
Source: Children's Hospital of Philadelphia

"Although crash risk is elevated for all newly licensed drivers, the study team found it is 62 percent higher for those with ADHD the first month after getting licensed, and 37 percent higher during the first four years after licensure, regardless of their age when licensed."

The operative words are, "regardless of age when first licensed,"

ADHD is associated with a significant increase in violence.

For a fact check and deeper look I refer the reader to:

Driving and Road Rage Associated with Attention Deficit Hyperactivity Disorder (ADHD): a Systematic Review.
Deshmukh, P., Patel, D.
Curr Dev Disord Rep 6, 241–247 (2019).
https://doi.org/10.1007/s40474-019-00183-9

How many patients must be treated for one patient to get better, the Number Needed to Treat, (NNT)?

How many patients must be treated for one patient to get worse, the number needed to harm one patient, (NNTH)?

Let us look at antipsychotic medications for an examination of the issues of efficacy, how effective is the medications, the number needed to treat, and the number needed to harm, and see if we can identify similar data for addicting medications.

Thorazine was the first synthesized in 1950 and marketed in France in 1951.

It was originally used for anesthesia.

However, it was soon noticed to improve the symptoms of schizophrenia and became the primary antipsychotic of its time.

It is still useful for schizophrenia, bipolar mania, aggression in children, for nausea and vomiting, insomnia, anxiety and pain.

One of the risks of Thorazine is that it is possible to have a ruptured appendix and die from peritonitis because the patient might not experience the pain that normally sends the patient to the hospital emergency room.

For a fact check, bibliography and more information I refer the reader to:

Fifty years chlorpromazine: a historical perspective
Thomas A Ban

Neuropsychiatr Dis Treat. 2007 Aug; 3(4): 495–500.
PMCID: PMC2655089
PMID: 19300578

"As early as 1956 it was determined that a single dose of 100mg of Thorazine or 25 mg of Thorazine three or four times a day is sufficient to resolve the psychosis of Acute Intermittent Porphyria."

"Thorazine does not cure Acute Intermittent Porphyria. It is not known by what mechanism Acute Intermittent Porphyria causes psychotic episodes that respond to Thorazine."

"It is speculated that because Thorazine binds to the D_2 dopamine receptors, the antipsychotic effect is due to blockade of the D_2 dopamine receptors."

"It is believed that hallucinations, delusions and paranoia of schizophrenia are due to hyperactivity of dopamine at D2 receptors in the mesolimbic pathway of the brain."

"D2 stimulators (agonists) include opiates, alcohol, nicotine, amphetamines, and cocaine. The use of opiates, alcohol, amphetamines, and cocaine are associated with psychotic episodes and aggression."

For fact checking and a more complete examination of the diagnosis and treatment of Schizophrenia I refer the reader to:
Schizophrenia A Diagnosis Looking for a Cause
Your Seventh Psychiatric Consultation
William Yee M.D., J.D.
Copyright Applied for 01/21/2020
Currently available from Amazon.

There has been extensive research on D_2 saturation and the treatment of schizophrenia.

Low doses of antipsychotic medications achieve effective saturation of D_2 receptors that causes a remission of symptoms.

Above this level of saturation extrapyramidal side effects that lead to Tardive Dyskinesia emerge.

Above the level that cause extrapyramidal side effects there is elevation of prolactin, gynecomastia and lactation in both males and females.

Past the first level there is no additional reduction of psychotic symptoms.

D_2 saturation at 65% yields a therapeutic effect.

D_2 saturation at 72% yields elevated prolactin levels, gynecomastia and lactation in both males and females.

D_2 saturation at 78% yields extrapyramydal symptoms and Tardive Dyskinesia, (EPS).

D_2 saturation above 65% does not appear to provide additional benefits in reducing psychotic symptoms and only causes gynecomastia with lactation in both men and women and at higher levels, Tardive Dyskinesia, (EPS).

The lowest effective dose the best practice.

Exceeding the lowest effective dose appears to cause serious side effects without a benefit according to research published as early as 2000.

See, "Relationship Between Dopamine D 2 Occupancy, Clinical Response, and Side Effects: A Double-Blind PET Study of First-Episode Schizophrenia," Shitij Kapur, M.D., Ph.D., F.R.C.P.C., Robert Zipursky, M.D., F.R.C.P.C., Corey Jones, B.A., Gary Remington, M.D., Ph.D., F.R.C.P.C., and Sylvain Houle, M.D., Ph.D., F.R.C.P.C. Am J Psychiatry 157:4, April 2000

Kapur recommends less than five milligrams of Haldol daily.

There have been advocates of high dose medications despite Kapur's research.

What is the best evidenced based practice?

I advocate for the lowest dose possible. I leave it to others to find the evidence supporting high doses of antipsychotic medications.

Schizophrenia is treated with individual, group and milieux therapies with the object of restoring a functional recovery.

A functional recovery is not an elimination of symptoms or "normal," functioning.

A functional recover is the ability to function effectively while having symptoms.

It is like being blind and being able to live.

The CATIE Schizophrenia Trial described the current state of the art of psychiatry.

The CATIE Schizophrenia Trial involved 1493 patients with schizophrenia treated with
olanzapine (7.5 to 30 mg per day),
perphenazine (8 to 32 mg per day),
quetiapine (200 to 800 mg per day),
or risperidone (1.5 to 6.0 mg per day)
Ziprasidone (40 to 160 mg per day)
for up to 18 months.

In the CATIE trial About 74 percent of patients discontinued their medication before 18 months

64 percent olanzapine,

75 percent perphenazine
82 percent quetiapine
74 percent risperidone
79 percent of those assigned to
ziprasidone.

The consensus among patients is that no
medication is the best choice based upon
the data above.

Another perspective is functional
recovery.

Examine the "Post by Former NIMH
Director Thomas Insel: Antipsychotics:
Taking the Long View," By Thomas Insel
on August 28, 2013.

Thomas R. Insel, M.D is credible by virtue
of the fact that he was Director of the
National Institute of Mental Health
(NIMH) from 2002-2015.

The literature and the pharmaceutical
industry warn of a decline in function
with each psychotic break. Dr. Insel
points to facts that suggest moderation in
the use of antipsychotic medication for
the best results.

Dr. Insel pointed out the fact that patients that were treated with antipsychotics and had a six-month remission and stopped the antipsychotics had a functional recovery rate of 40.4 percent after seven years.

Dr. Insel pointed out the fact that patients that were treated with antipsychotics and had a six-month remission and continued the antipsychotics had a functional recovery rate of only 17.6 percent after seven years.

Dr. Insel points out that a functional recovery is often better served by stopping the antipsychotic medications and focusing on alternative treatments.

It is speculated that flat affect, lack of psychosocial motivation and engagement, and other negative symptoms of schizophrenia may be due to under stimulation of the D_1 receptors.

Although it is known that D2 receptors are involved in hallucinations, delusions, and paranoia. That does not yield the cause of schizophrenia. There are many causes of hallucinations, delusions and paranoia.

There are many inconsistencies in the medical literature.

Given the context above let us look at the use of Clozaril, Adderall, Ambien, and Xanax for the treatment of psychosis, ADHD, insomnia and anxiety.

The Gold Standard for antipsychotic medications is Clozaril/Clozapine. Let us look at the FDA Label for Clozaril/Clozapine in terms of efficacy, duration of treatment, risks and benefits.

Then, let us compare Adderall, Ambien and Xanax FDA labels in terms of duration of treatment, risks and benefits.

Since clozapine is considered the "Gold Standard" as the most effective medication for schizophrenia, let's examine the side effects of clozapine as reported in the FDA Label for Clozapine.

Clozapine has a black box warning for:

"AGRANULOCYTOSIS that can result in death; ORTHOSTATIC HYPOTENSION that can result in falls and injuries, BRADYCARDIA that can be life threatening, AND SYNCOPE that can result in falls and injuries; SEIZURE that may result in injury and death; MYOCARDITIS that may result in death, AND CARDIOMYOPATHY that can result in death; INCREASED MORTALITY IN ELDERLY PATIENTS WITH DEMENTIA RELATED PSYCHOSIS"

Clozapine has other serious side effects that include QT prolongation, Torsades de Pointes and other ventricular arrhythmias including cardiac arrest that can cause death.

Clozapine can cause a metabolic syndrome that includes hyperglycemia, dyslipidemia, and obesity that leads to Type II diabetes and all the complications of diabetes.

Clozapine can cause Neuroleptic Malignant Syndrome (NMS) which includes high fever, muscle rigidity, altered mental status, autonomic instability, irregular pulse, unstable blood pressure, tachycardia, diaphoresis, and cardiac dysrhythmias that can result in kidney failure and death.

Clozapine can cause pulmonary embolism and deep vein thrombosis which often leads to death.

Clozapine can cause anticholinergic effects resulting in acute open angle glaucoma, blindness, delirium, constipation, prostatic hypertrophy, difficulty urination, urinary retention, renal failure and bowel obstruction, and death.

Clozapine can cause tardive dyskinesia which can manifest irreversible motor movements at rest.

Clozapine can cause many other side effects and the FDA Clozaril Label should be reviewed directly before starting the medication.

The Clozaril FDA Label indicates that ten studies were pooled comparing Clozaril to Thorazine:

"The median duration of CLOZARIL and chlorpromazine exposure was 45 days and 38 days, respectively."

For all of this risk the FDA label states that 30% of the patients that received the Clozapine had a 20% reduction in symptoms.

That translates to treating four patients for only one patient to benefit by a 20% reduction in the symptoms of schizophrenia due to the use of Clozaril.

"Patients treated with CLOZARIL had a statistically significant longer delay in the time to recurrent suicidal behavior in comparison with olanzapine."

Antipsychotics are not much different in efficacy. Only small differences in benefit as compared to large differences in side effects. It is reasonable to conclude that sedating medications such as Clozaril, Zyprexa and Chlorpromazine all reduce impulsive behaviors, aggression and suicide.

Activating antipsychotic medications such as Abilify are known to increase impulsive behaviors including gambling and would be contraindicated in the suicidal patient.

Let us look at Ambien as an example of an addicting sleeping pill.

FDA adds Boxed Warning for risk of serious injuries caused by sleepwalking with certain prescription insomnia medicines. The following medications merit your attention: eszopiclone (Lunesta), zaleplon (Sonata), and zolpidem (Ambien, Ambien CR, Edluar, Intermezzo, Zolpimist) when compared to other prescription medicines used for sleep.

More than seventy percent of patients on Ambien continue Ambien after fourteen days although it is known to lose effect after fourteen days.

For a fact check and entry into the literature I refer the reader to:

"77% of patients ignore FDA safety recommendations for Ambien"
Moore TJ, et al. JAMA Intern Med. 2018; doi:10.1001/jamainternmed.2018.3031. July 19, 2018.

Amphetamine and methamphetamine are structurally similar with similar mechanism of action. The primary difference is the percentage that penetrates the blood brain barrier to enter the brain.

More methamphetamine gets into the brain than amphetamine.

More heroine gets into the brain then morphine.

If you increase the dose of the amphetamine and morphine you obtain the same effects, side effects, addictions and physiologic and injuries to the brain as with methamphetamine and heroine

Let us look at amphetamines like Adderall.

Long term exposure leads to addiction and with addiction rebound symptoms when the amphetamines are withdrawn.

Amphetamines are used to treat ADHD and ADD, but the brain is so complex it is not known exactly what the problem is. Therefore, the mode of therapeutic action in Attention Deficit Hyperactivity Disorder (ADHD) is not known.

Let us look at pharmacokinetics of amphetamines.
The peek blood level is achieved about three hours after taking the medication and the half-life is about ten hours.

It takes about four half-lives to eliminate 95% of the amphetamine from the blood.

The "rush" that drug addicts seek when using drugs is experienced during that first three hours when the blood level and presumably the brain level of amphetamines is rising to its peak. The letdown is that forty-hour period when the blood level is falling.

During that forty-hours that it takes for

the medication to clear form the blood, eating and sleeping are impaired which can stunt the growth of a child.

That is often the reason that patients on amphetamines ask for sleeping pills. The amphetamines keep them up at night.

The average person starts hallucinating after 72 consecutive hours of total sleep deprivation. Hallucinations and psychosis can develop with prolonged periods of partial sleep deprivation.

Even the most skilled expert in ADHD diagnosis and treatment cannot say with absolute certainty that a given patient has ADHD for the simple fact that it is a collection of symptoms that can have many causes.

Examine the official FDA Label for Adderall:

"Special Diagnostic Considerations Specific etiology of this syndrome is unknown, and there is no single diagnostic test. Adequate diagnosis requires the use not only of medical but of special psychological, educational, and social resources. Learning may or may not be impaired. The diagnosis must be based upon a complete history and evaluation of the child and not solely on the presence of the required number of DSM-IV® characteristics."

The use of amphetamines for ADHD is a last resort after alternative interventions are utilized.

Again, examine the FDA Label for Adderall:

"Need for Comprehensive Treatment Program Adderall® is indicated as an integral part of a total treatment program for ADHD that may include other measures (psychological, educational, social) for patients with this syndrome. Drug treatment may not be indicated for all children with this syndrome. Stimulants are not intended for use in the child who exhibits symptoms secondary to environmental factors and/or other primary psychiatric disorders, including psychosis.

Appropriate educational placement is essential and psychosocial intervention is often helpful. When remedial measures alone are insufficient, the decision to prescribe stimulant medication will depend upon the physician's assessment of the chronicity and severity of the child's symptoms."

The problem with all addicting medications, including amphetamines is that they are only useful for the short term.

With addiction, the reduction of pain, insomnia, anxiety, and symptoms of ADHD attenuate, and the patient is taking the medication because of addiction and to avoid the rebound.

What is rebound?

Rebound is the exaggerated pain, anxiety, insomnia, and ADHD symptoms when the addicting medications are stopped.

After addiction the original pain, anxiety,

insomnia and ADHD are worse than before the medication was started. Watch videos on youtube of people going through alcohol and opiate withdrawal to see how severe the pain, anxiety and insomnia are during rebound.

The rebound of methamphetamines is hypersomnia and anergy that mask the rebound of the ADHD symptoms.

There is no scientific basis for denying the rebound of ADHD symptoms after addiction and withdrawal.

Again, examine the FDA label for Adderall:

"Long-Term Use The effectiveness of Adderall® for long-term use has not been systematically evaluated in controlled trials. Therefore, the physician who elects to use Adderall® for extended periods should periodically reevaluate the long-term usefulness of the drug for the individual patient."

There is no incentive for the manufacturer of Adderall to examine the long-term adverse effect and side effect of Adderall, knowing that addiction and rebound are inevitable.

The average person confuses the suppression of rebound after long term use of Adderall with a therapeutic effect, rather than a masking of an antitherapeutic effect or pathological effect.

I have been practicing medicine and psychiatry since 1972.

I have been an expert witness as a board-certified psychiatrist in probate, civil and criminal cases in state and federal courts in Michigan, Indiana, Kentucky and California.

As a psychiatrist I have listened to hundreds of patients tell me about their childhood trauma and PTSD. Most of the trauma occurred in chaotic families created by drug addicted parents, who were often antisocial or borderline personalities or both.

In view of all that precedes I make the following recommendations.

Because of accidents and road rage associated with ADHD I recommend against handgun permits, licenses to fly and operating dangerous machinery for people with ADHD.

I recommend against the use of Adderall and other psychostimulants for patients under stress as Adderall increases the risk of paranoia, delusions and violent behavior during periods of stress.

In view of dissociative states, addiction and rebound insomnia I recommend against the use of Ambien for people under stress, depressed or with suicidal tendencies.

I also recommend against the use of Ambien when patients are starting antidepressants because of the black box warning about suicide with the use of antidepressants.

I recommend against the use of Ambien and other sleeping pills because of dissociative states when the patient has a handgun permit or is licensed to fly or engages in other risky activities, or is depressed and suicidal

I recommend for the use of Clozaril, Zyprexa and Chlorpromazine for patients taking antidepressants when suicidal symptoms are present as frontal lobe executive functions and impulses that plan and execute suicide attempts are suppressed by Clozaril, Zyprexa and Chlorpromazine.

Clozaril, Zyprexa and Chlorpromazine reduce suicide risk during the early period when antidepressant medications increase energy before the reduction of depression.

Thank you for your time and attention.
William R. Yee, M.D., J.D.
Board Certified Psychiatrist
Practicing psychiatry without interruption in Michigan, Indiana, Kentucky, California and Texas since 1972, at your service.
I am here to do no harm and help if I can.

"Preexisting text," includes names of symptoms, medical illnesses, medications, people, corporations, law cases, statutes, text of statutes, the titles of articles and books, the content of articles and books cited.

My copyright claim is a clam to the "original text," which is my personal experiences as described in the text above and my commentary on the preexisting text listed above.